COSMETOLOGY SPECIALTIES

for the

BEDRIDDEN PATIENT

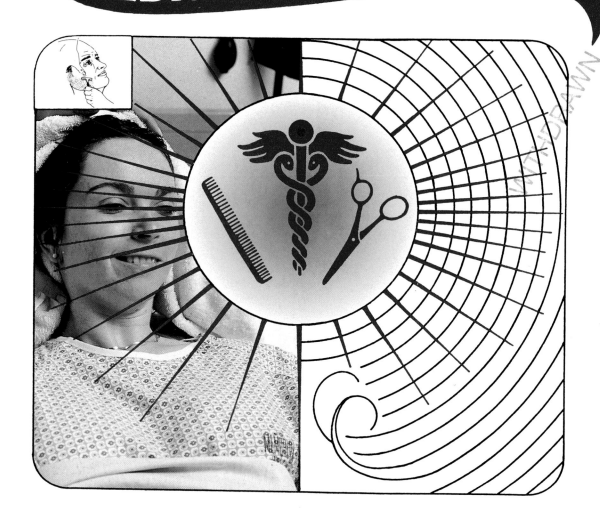

Noëlla Charest-Papagno

COSMETOLOGY SPECIALTIES

for the

BEDRIDDEN PATIENT

Noëlla Charest-Papagno, L.C., A.S.

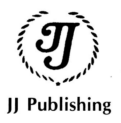

JJ Publishing

Cover & Illustrations by Jose Chavarry

First Edition 1996

Publisher's Cataloging in Publication

Charest-Papagno, Noëlla.
  Cosmetology specialties for the bedridden patient / Noëlla Charest-Papagno.
  p. cm.
  Includes index.
  Preassigned LCCN: 95-78324
  ISBN 0-9604610-6-X

  1. Beauty culture. 2. Sick--Services for. 3. Handicapped--Services for. I. Title.

TT957.C46 1996   646.7'024'0816
                                     QBI96-20295

JJ Publishing, 1312 Arthur Street
Hollywood, Florida 33019 (954) 929-3559
Printed in the United States of America

ACKNOWLEDMENTS

My sincere gratitude is owed to the following people who so generously offered information and support:

* The Honorable John B. Anderson

* Frederic S. Herold, M.D.

* Guery Davis, PhD, Florida Department of Education at Tallahassee, Florida

* Karen Freeman, Patient Care Manager, Vistas Innovative Hospice Care, Inc. Aventura Hospital and Medical Center at Aventura, Florida

* Judith Joseph, The School Board of Broward County, Florida

* The Broward Community College at Davie, Florida, my Alma Mater

Noëlla

DEDICATED TO

⁕ Members of my family---especially my daughter, Jane (RN), who inspired me to write this book.

⁕ Medical professionals and assistive personnel that deliver patient care in health facilities and private residences in order to help the bedridden regain their health, independence and/or make their lives as comfortable as possible.

⁕ Those in the beauty salon industry who have made cosmetology a respected art and science and also for the important services provided by them over these many years.

PREFACE

This book was written to provide in sufficient details essential information to enable medical professionals and assistive personnel, salon professionals and the bedridden patient's family member(s) to meet the cosmetology needs of the bedridden. Using methods described in this publication, you will learn how to prepare the bedridden and you will be provided the methodology created especially for this work. Cosmetology specialties can now be performed at hospitals, nursing homes, private residences with limited work space and facilities available to each bedridden patient.

The author's wealth of experience, based on many years as a practicing cosmetologist, has developed the necessary credentials and knowledge. This has enabled her to address the issues involved in meeting the cosmetology needs of this segment of our population that, for the most part, has been neglected. The innovative and specialized procedures are as follows:

* A 20 minute treatment that consists of brushing, washing, rinsing the hair and scalp of the bedridden
* Trimming the bedridden's hair in, or out-of-bed
* 4 selected hairstyles
* Mini facial
* Mini manicure and pedicure
* Haircoloring
* Partial permanent waving
* Care of wigs and hairpieces
* Shaving (male face)
* Shaping of the beard, mustache, and eyebrows

DISCLAIMER

The author and publisher have made considerable effort to insure that the material contained in this book is as accurate as possible and conforms to standards of contemporary cosmetology. In as much as the bulk of the information contained herein pertains to, and is directed at the bedridden i.e. persons with serious disorders or medical problem(s), the risk of injury to both provider and the patient as a result of poor judgement, human error etc., is substantially greater than for healthy individuals provided these same services. The author and publisher assume no responsibility for any injury suffered by either the patient(s) or provider(s) in connection with use of material contained in this book.

TABLE OF CONTENTS

FOREWORD

This Foreword is written for my friend Noëlla Charest-Papagno as an affectionate tribute to her determined and long-standing effort to make a distinctive contribution to her chosen profession. Into this slender volume, she has poured her intense interest in caring for people whose needs would otherwise be unserved.

Noëlla has outlined very carefully and with precision, the steps that can be taken to meet cosmetology needs of the bed-ridden patient and people with disabilities who continue to take pride in their appearance. Self-esteem is an essential ingredient to any person, whether well or in ill health. For the sake of self-respect, there endures in the vast majority of people a deep desire to look their best.

With the aging of the American population, long-term care needs will dramatically expand in many different areas. The author has carved out a special niche for health care professionals and other caregivers to help meet those needs. This is a book that should open the eyes of the cosmetology salon professionals to the role that they too can play. The fact that the author took the time to research and write this book shows how much she cares for people and for her chosen profession.

John B. Anderson

Former member of the United States Congress
Independent Candidate for President 1980
Currently President of The World Federalist Association

Obviously, cosmetology needs of the acutely ill patient are of little concern in certain situations e.g. a bedridden soon after surgery, during periods of intensive care or during circumstances where the clinical objective is one of patient survival. Chronically ill patients in institutions such as nursing homes, in private residences and hospices*, are usually being treated medically by a physician along with support from registered nurses, other qualified medical professionals, assistive personnel and in many cases members of the patient's family and/or friends.

Even in cases where a patient requests some form of cosmetology, it is essential that the patient's personal PHYSICIAN and/or the patient's assigned nurse be consulted before any services are rendered to the individual---to ensure that the procedures employed, such as washing the hair, are not incompatible with the medical condition or pose any additional risk to the patient. Although all patients have a right to privacy, anyone providing cosmetology should be made aware of any relevant medical condition that can be exacerbated or even induce an adverse response in the patient. For example, washing the hair of patients with spinal cord or scalp injuries should be attempted only if approved by the patient's PHYSICIAN and only if any movement of the patient is made by or under the direction of a qualified medical professional. Also, if it is determined that the patient has a perforated ear drum, use of ear plugs should be considered, to prevent anything e.g. water from entering the ear. Finally, it is reasonable for the person performing cosmetology services, to be made aware of lesions (sores), so it can be decided if these present a risk of <u>serious</u> infection to you, the provider.

For purposes of simplification, in this publication, the registered nurse, (RN) and licensed practical/vocational nurse, (LPN/ LVN) in charge of the patient will be designated as the "ASSIGNED NURSE". The assistive personnel e.g. patient care and nursing assistant, home health aide, orderly and/or volunteer will be referred to as "ASSISTANT". The family member(s) and/ or the bedridden's close friend who serve in place of a family member will be referred to also as the "ASSISTANT". Finally providing services for the various cosmetology specialties will be refered to as CosmeCare.

* Details of Hospice and this special kind of caregiving is included in the Appendix "What Is Hospice"

THE AUTHOR SPEAKS TO THE READER

The scope for this book is not merely a "how to" treatise. It is more of a philosophy on satisfying a great need for bedridden people with their inability to avail themselves of their lifelong habit and ritual of periodic cosmetology care. My background in Medical Assisting Technology and the love of cosmetology presented me with the drive to develop step-by-step techniques that take into consideration the tenderness and sensitivity requirements of the bedridden individual.

The book contains descriptions for preparation of the bedridden, the proper way to move the patient (and precautions) when required, stages in techniques where medical advice is required and where help of an ASSISTANT is needed to move the patient. Disorders of the hair, skin and nails and the need for Universal Precaution are addressed. Also details on the supplies needed for providing each of these services.

I would like to hear from those of you who have purchased this book and have adopted these cosmetology methods. I would like to learn of your success (hopefully no failure) in providing services to bedridden patients and to inform me of any inconveniences and/or interesting experiences. If you have any questions or would like to have further discussion e.g., explanations of material contained in this book---write to me and I will do my best to answer any questions you may have and give suggestions that you might find helpful.

Author of:
Handbook of Desairology
for Cosmetologists
Servicing Funeral Homes

JJ Publishing
1312 Arthur St.; Dept. E
Hollywood, Florida 33019

A noted Neurologist reported that procedures involving arching or twisting a person's neck in order to wash the hair or rinse and neutralize a permanent, <u>increases the risk of stroke or lesser forms of brain damage</u>. The hazards are increased in older people and young adults with high blood pressure, diabetes and those having hidden malfunction of a main artery (vertebral arteries) that lie in the spinal column (actually there are two) and supplies blood to the brain; shown are <u>normal arteries </u>(a).

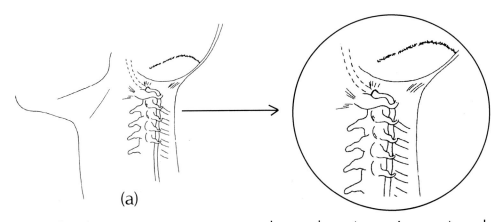

(a)

These findings were presented at the American Academy of Neurology Annual Meeting in 1994. The Academy called for those salon professionals with clients at increased risk to be alert for what could happen during those procedures. The increased risk was attributed to several factors, (1) because these arteries lie next to the bones of the neck, the arteries are *stretched* and may be compressed when the neck is *twisted* e.g. chin to shoulder or bent in an extreme manner; further with age, these same arteries also tend to become clogged with fatty deposits and/or have arthritic changes in the bones of their necks that give rise to bony spikes on the cervical vertebrae.

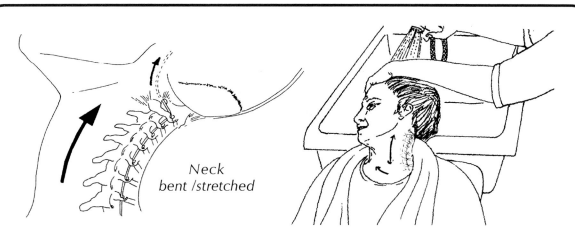

Neck
bent /stretched

Reduced blood flow can result in dizziness, nausea, loss of balance, numbness on one side of the body and/or perhaps a stroke. The Neurologist suggested that there is a need to develop safer hairwashing and rinsing methods. The methodology recommended in this publication has made it a point to be cognizant of this problem i.e. improper misalignment of the head and neck, also illustrated below.

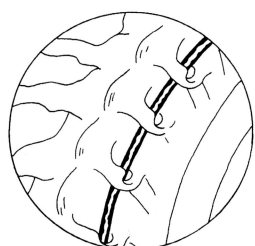

Fatty deposits

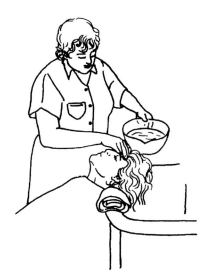

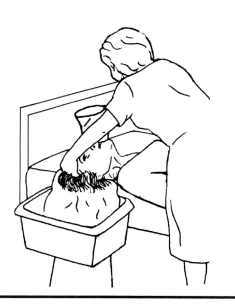

WHO ARE THE BEDRIDDEN?

The elderly, when sick, do not comprise the only group of patients restricted to a bed, although they undoubtedly represent the largest segment of the bedridden population. There are countless cases of younger persons, who are not ambulatory and are therefore, restricted to a bed for extended periods of time---at home or in a health care facility (related to either an illness or as the result of an accident). There are thousands of individuals who are not in a dedicated facility, yet are incapable of meeting these CosmeCare needs for themselves e.g. upper body neuromuscular deficits, joint disease, or those who loose or have limited use of a hand(s) and/or an arm(s).

It is not uncommon for individuals that are bedridden to suffer some, if not significant degrees of mental depression. CosmeCare is therapeutic for the bedridden because it relaxes both the body and the mind and reduces pain and stress. There is hardly a bedridden woman who does not appreciate that a clean attractively styled hair and properly "made-up" face or even manicured nails, can give them a needed lift in spirit and self-esteem. It is only natural that a bedridden patient likes to hear from others---that they are "looking better".

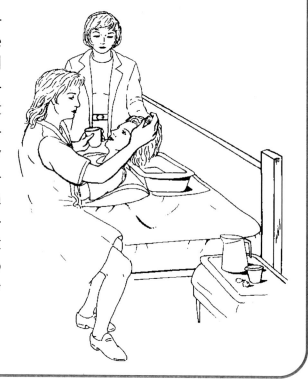

Some planning, especially in medical facilities, is necessary to minimize disruptions and wasting of time for you, the bedridden and those directly involved in patient care e.g., nurses and assistive personnel. Check with the patient's ASSIGNED NURSE by phone to verify that the patient will be available, and well enough, prior to your visit. You should inform the ASSIGNED NURSE in sufficient details of the service(s) you intend to render, the approximate time required for completion of these procedures, and that the order for the appointment has been cleared with the patient's personal physician at the time it was initially requested. Upon your arrival, go directly to the nurse's station on the patient's floor and check with the ASSIGNED NURSE to determine whether any new orders were written by the physician that would be important for you to be aware of.

Let the NURSE introduce you to the patient whenever possible. If she/he is not able to do this, go to where the patient is located and identify the bedridden for yourself. Ask the patient to tell you their name---do not offer the name. They may nod or say "yes" and she/he may not be the correct patient for the requested CosmeCare services. Check the patient's identity bracelet on their arm or leg. This should correctly identify the individual and whether or not they are alert and oriented. Tell the patient your name unless the patient already knows and/or recognizes you. Be friendly and have a caring attitude. Ask the patient if they have allergies or sensitivities to any hair, skin or nail products.

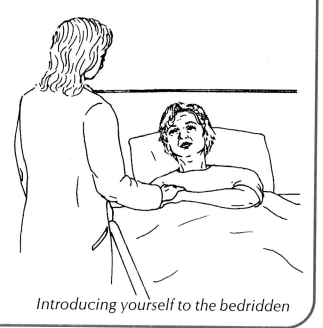

Introducing yourself to the bedridden

This is in addition to questioning the NURSE---it pays to be careful. The following suggestions are important before, during and after CosmeCare procedures:

✳ <u>Always</u> have a qualified ASSISTANT move or position the patient for you.

✳ If the patient feels comfortable about services that she/he, or the FAMILY requested, then you can begin checking and assembling the necessary supplies. Place supplies in the strategic locations where they will be easily accessible, when needed. Involve the patient (wherever possible) in any discussion related to your services so that the individual is comfortable with your proposed plan. Ask questions pertaining to the services that can be answered in simple terms e.g., yes or no. If the patient does not interact, talk about your plan out loud, anyway. It may be that the patient can understand and is just not able to respond or may be medicated.

✳ To prevent patients from falling out-of-bed, lift the bed rail into upward position if you have to leave the patient or if you leave the room unattended.

✳ Lower only one bed rail at a time---never both.

✳ Allow sufficient time for completing each procedure(s) and the proper cleaning of supplies and workplace when finished.

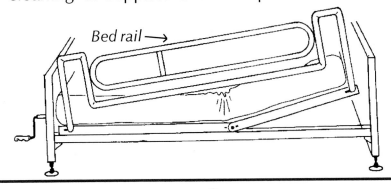

Bed rail →

✳ For the bedridden who have not had any hair care for pro-
tracted periods of time and the process of washing hair <u>per se</u>
are both factors that can result in knotted or tangled hair. Clear-
ing the tangles should be accomplished without pulling or using
excessive force on the hair.

✳ Logistically, it makes good sense to have the patient remain in
bed for washing the hair in view of the amount of time required
for this procedure and the enjoyment and the relaxation it provides. Where the patient is able, or encouraged, to get out-of-
bed, the advantage of trimming or rinsing the hair out-of-bed are
obvious---psychologically, if not medically. Thus, in most all
cases, trimming the patient's hair is carried out after washing.

✳ Always use one of your hands to monitor the temperature of the air
coming from the hair dryer to insure that the patient's hair or scalp
are not exposed to excessive heat---should the patient be medicated
and/or insensitive to normal thermal stimuli or pain.

✳ For medical, as well as usual cosmetic reasons, you may be asked
to remove artificial nails from a patient's nail(s). If the finger(s) or
nails appear abnormal (inflamed, red or infected) you should inform
the ASSIGNED NURSE before proceeding.

✳ Depending on the facility and medical history, there may be instances where the application of nail polish or cosmetics may be
desired and may be requested.

✳ For those who prefer an electric shaver, direction for use of this
device is obvious and unnecessary. Trimming a beard or a mustache can be performed without an electric clipper---however, it
takes longer with a comb and scissors.

✳ Make a list of all the needed supplies and allow sufficient time for
cleaning.

UNIVERSAL PRECAUTIONS

Practicing Universal Precaution means being careful to prevent injury or placing both the bedridden patient, and you, at increased risk. When providing CosmeCare, you should consider employment of barriers such as, latex disposal gloves, an apron and/or face (surgical) masks. Since a high proportion of the bedridden population may have a reduced or impaired immune system as a result of the disease process itself and/or the therapy employed to treat the disease, it is important that all supplies used be either disposable or adequately washed with soapy water, then treated with antiseptics/disinfectants before and after use on a patient. This level of sanitation is needed to prevent additional medical burden to the patient, as well as preventing the spread of microorganisms e.g. from patient-to-patient or patient to you. All combs and hair brushes as well as other items that come in direct contact with the patient should be placed in clean, plastic bags and sealed until needed. When your services are completed all items used should be returned to the bag and the bag sealed. All supplies whether for disposal or to be reused, should be retreated with an antiseptic before reusing or disposal. To insure that the hands are clean the following procedure can be followed:

1. Wet hands and apply antiseptic soap, rub hands together to work up a lather by applying friction; interlace your fingers; clean around and under the nails; then, extend the washing to include well beyond the wrists.

2. Rinse the hands with running tap water held directly over the sink; towel dry; then rinse the hands with a small amount of 70% isopropyl alcohol (U.S.P.) or alcohol sponge; allow the hands to dry.

CHAPTER ONE

Hair

We are all very familiar with hair but it is helpful to briefly review the nature of these structures. The type, pattern and growth of hair differs in male and female individuals and is based in large part on the level of androgens (male sex hormones) and also differs amongst different races as determined by heredity (genes).

STRUCTURE - Hair grows by forming new cells at the base of the hair (root) in specialized tissue or hair follicle. These new cells push the older cells toward the surface of the skin, only to die, become keratinized and become part of the hair shaft. A human scalp hair grows about 0.5 inches per month for two or four years at which time it falls out and a new hair begins to grow. Shorter hairs on the body tend to be replaced sooner e.g. eye lashes grow for perhaps three to five months before the hair is replaced with a new one. A great many factors can influence the rate of hair growth including age, diet, disease, hormonal levels (endocrine glands), as well as many factors that are yet unknown. In some cases of hair loss, hair follicles remain viable for years without any observable hair growth. The hair follicle ends in a papilla, a highly vascular (rich in blood vessels) structure that supplies nutrients for hair growth.

Hair color (like skin color) is influenced by genetic factors that determines the amount of melanin that is deposited in the hair as it grows. In the latter case, reduced, or the absence of melanin, results in gray or white hair. It should be of no great surprise to anyone that the color of hair can be markedly changed by use of a variety of different chemical agents e.g. haircolor, and hydrogen peroxide, as well as natural changes that alter melanin production. Studies show that cells in the hair structure tends to grow at unequal rates to give shapes that vary from round to flattened. Thus, the flatter the hair, the wavier or curlier it becomes.

The various parts of a hair are provided in the illustrations showing (1) a hair in a cross section. Magnification of a hair shows specialized cells, of which 90% are found in the cortex (the mid-central part). It also reveals a medulla (the center) and the cuticle (the outer sheath) (2) section showing the hair follicle, hair shaft, root, papilla and bulb.

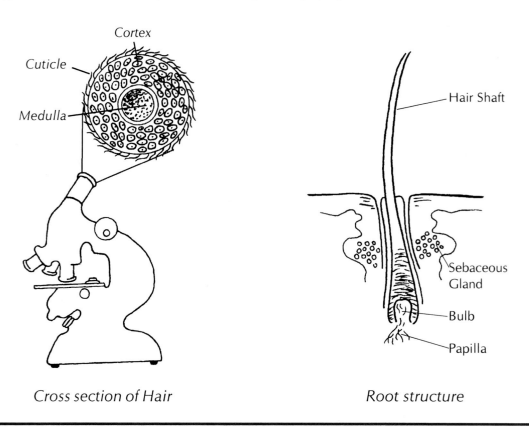

Cross section of Hair   *Root structure*

Exposure to the sun, improper use of chemicals (including hair products) can result in structural damage that results in hair that is easily broken. Neglect of the scalp and/or people's physical and medical conditions, may be contributing factors resulting in damaged hair. Hair is considered overly damaged when it is rough and harsh to the touch, or has lost its elasticity. When washed, damaged hair, (especially the ends) may sometimes feel spongy and mats easily. A comparison of normal and damaged hair is illustrated below. Also, the structural integrity and quality of hair may be compromised as a result of the patient's medical condition or its treatment e.g. radiation. Even ordinary handling of hair can lead to unwarranted hair loss in these cases.

✳. <u>Suggested Course of Action</u> - Trim the ends of the hair if requested. Refer to "Treating Tangled Hair" in Chapter 2; then apply a "leave in" conditioner; proceed with selected hairstyle or blow dry the hair. Observe warnings when using the blow dryer.

Magnification of Hair Cuticles

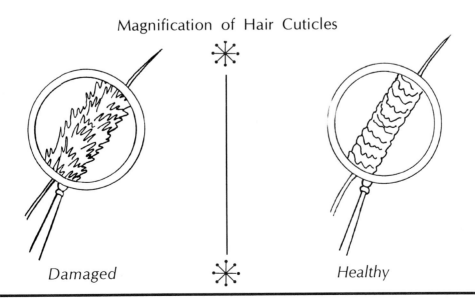

Damaged   Healthy

When unfamiliar lesions e.g. sores, are encountered, consider delaying the washing of the hair and scalp, perming or haircoloring the hair until a medical diagnoses and treatment (where possible) has been carried out in order to prevent further injury or spread of infectious agent(s). This delay is more important for those who are less likely to be proficient in use of basic sanitary protocols, (Universal Precaution) and/or recognizing the lesion(s). The following is a list of some of the common hair and scalp disorders.

DANDRUFF (Pityriasis) - This condition results from the accumulation of cells shed from the scalp, that appear on the hair---the more rapidly the cells are shed, the more the dandruff. Some authorities hold that long neglected dandruff can lead to hair loss. Long standing dandruff can promote the growth of microorganisms e.g. yeast, fungus, bacteria etc. Dandruff is thought to be due to factors such as diet, emotional stress, and glandular disturbances, lack of nerve stimulation and uncleaned or improperly cleaned hair and scalp. The two principal types of dandruff are as follows:

a). *Dry Dandruff* (Pityriasis Capitis Simplex) The cells are seen a thick white scales, usually attached to the scalp, or scattered loosely throughout the hair. Occasionally, dandruff is so heavy that some of it will be easily noticed on the clothing at the shoulders (with some embarrassment to the person).

b). *Greasy* (or waxy) *Dandruff* (Pityriasis Steatoides) In this condition the cells shed from the scalp are mixed with sebum from the sebaceous glands causing the cells to stick or or adhere to the scalp. If greasy dandruff is pulled from the scalp, oozing of sebum may follow.

WASHING THE HAIR AND SCALP CAN CAUSE A DAN-DRUFF-LIKE CONDITION - There are instances where improper washing of hair and scalp can actually produce encrusted dandruff in *areas* of the scalp. This condition arises when shampoo is applied directly from the bottle onto the scalp (without first diluting the product with wa-

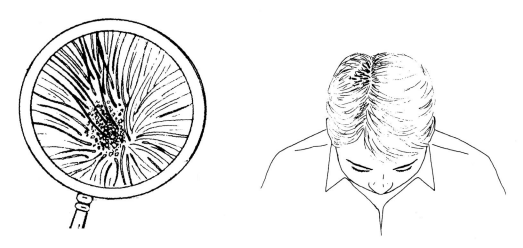

Accumulated shampoo and soap residue

ter) or bar soap is used for washing the hair and scalp and then is followed by *insufficient dispersing* and *rinsing*. When this practice is repeated again and again, shampoo or soap accumulates in the targeted area(s), dries and results in patches of dandruff like material. This can cause the scalp to become very irritated.

✳ <u>Suggested</u> <u>Course</u> <u>of</u> <u>Action</u>: Do not use a comb or hair brush to loosen or remove encrusted "dandruff" attached to the scalp. **DARA⁺R** is recommended initially then on a regular basis once the accumulated residue are removed.

HEAD LICE (Pediculosis Capitis) - This is an infestation involving the hair and scalp (although infestation of other parts of the body can occur). The lice live directly (feed) on the host and are transmitted by personal contact and/or by using objects such as combs, hair brushes, hats or head scarfs contaminated with lice or ova (egg). An inspection of the scalp (preferably with a magnifying lens) reveals small ovoid grayish-white ova, "nits", attached or

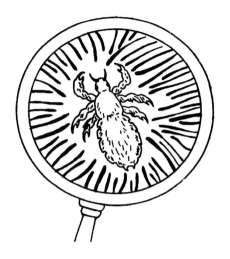

fixed to the hair shaft that are not easily dislodged. These ova are observed more frequently than the adult louse. Itching can be severe, sometimes leading to a secondary bacterial infection.

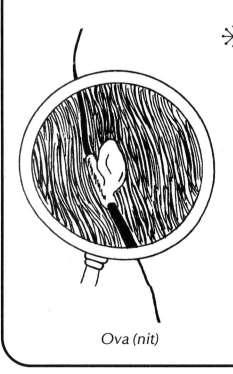

Ova (nit)

✳ <u>Suggested</u> <u>Course</u> <u>of</u> <u>Action</u>: Before any attempts are made to rid the patient of these parasites, the **ASSIGNED NURSE** at the facility, or the patient's **FAMILY**, must be made aware of the infestation so that appropriate delousing actions can be taken. With proper consent of a physician, prescribed or over-the-counter parasiticides in the form of a shampoo or lotion purchased from a pharmacy, can be used to rid patients of these parasites.

The hair and scalp should be retreated and examined after 10 days to be sure the patient is free of parasites or ova. Again, when in doubt, a magnifying lens can be helpful in differentiating ordinary cellular debris from ova. Proceed with CosmeCare after the lice are removed and approval is obtained.

PSORIASIS - This is a common chronic and recurrent skin disease involving the scalp and other areas of the body including nails. The cause is not known. In the scalp the lesions are well defined, dry, silvery and shiny scales. If the scale is removed a tiny amount of blood may appear. Since it is a chronic disease that is not contagious, it would be rare that the patient would not be aware of their having this disease and make it known to you (if they were lucid).

Suggested Course of Action: The patient usually has a prescribed ointment (which if directed by the patient or the **ASSIGNED NURSE**, is applied according to product's instruction). Proceed with Cosme-Care; omit brushing the hair, if requested.

BALDNESS (Alopecia) - This is a term used to describe partial or complete loss of hair. It may result from hormone imbalance, genetic factors, aging, diet, and from local or systemic diseases. The hair loss in Alopecia is not to be confused with hair loss that occurs

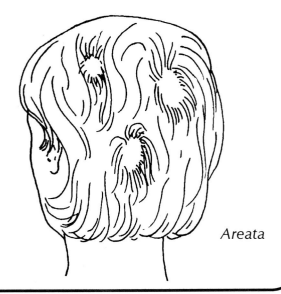

Areata

17

normally as the hair ages and is replaced. Alopecia can be classified as follows:

   a). *Areata:* Sudden hair loss in circumscribed areas or patches in the absence/obvious skin or systemic disease.

   b). *Toxic:* Usually temporary---after fever, cytotoxic agents (cancer chemotherapy); a large number of drugs and chemical agents.

   c). *Totalis:* General loss of scalp or body hair.

   d). *Universalis:* Total loss of hair all over the body.

✳ <u>Suggested</u> <u>Course</u> <u>of</u> <u>Action:</u> Obviously, there is little, if anything that can be done by you for Alopecia Totalis and Universalis---proceed with other CosmeCare procedures if requested.

TICK(S) - These are small parasites that become imbedded (bite) into tissue and draw blood from the host to feed; they attach to humans (and animals) and are found less frequently in the scalp and hair than in other parts of the body.

✳ <u>Suggested</u> <u>Course</u> <u>of</u> <u>Action:</u> If observed, notify the ASSIGNED NURSE (do not try to remove the insect) and proceed with CosmeCare after the tick(s) are removed and approval is obtained.

CYST (Steatoma) - This is a benign mass that is found on the skin (and scalp), it involves the sebaceous (oil) glands---resulting from accumulation of viscous matter (often foul smelling). Also referred to as a wen.

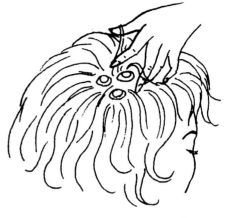
Cysts

✳ Suggested Course of Action: This lesion should be left to qualified medical professionals. With careful handling of the scalp, CosmeCare can be carried out, if permitted.

RINGWORM OF THE SCALP (Tinea Capitis) - This is a contagious condition that can become epidemic in children. It is a superficial fungus infection of the scalp and/or hair. It is characterized by round grayish patch(s), that become prominent with red spots at the opening of the follicles.
The patch(s) usually contain spores and a few mycelia, sometimes in rings, enlarge or coalesce until the entire scalp can be infected as shown; the hair involved becomes lusterless, brittle, lifeless and breaks off or falls outs.

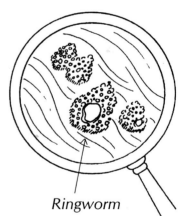
Ringworm

✳ Suggested Course of Action: Treatment should be left to qualified medical professionals and CosmeCare can be instituted only after successful therapy.

WART(S) (Verrucae) - These elevations on the surface of the scalp are the result of viral infections of the skin. The scalp lesion often resembling a "cauliflower".

✳ Suggested Course of Action: These abnormalities should be left to qualified medical professional for treatment. With careful handling of the scalp, CosmeCare can probably be carried out.

Tumor(s) - During routine CosmeCare, you may find overlooked masses or tumors on the scalp. It is conceivable that the tumor observed is a local growth or it can represent the spread of a malignant tumor from a distant site. In any case, it is not your place to make any statement that can be cause for anxiety in the bedridden but it is important that the presence of a mass be made known to the ASSIGNED NURSE in charge of the patient's care.

✳ Suggested Course of Action: Diagnoses and treatment should be left to qualified medical professionals. CosmeCare can usually be carried out, if permitted.

CHAPTER TWO

The Dᴀʀᴀ⁺ʀ Method Of Washing The Hair And Scalp

In general people tend to view washing of hair as an enjoyable and essential part of daily living. Healthy individuals take this pleasurable activity for granted. When people are ill, however, these activities are less likely to be available or rendered.

A person's hair and scalp when bedridden tend to accumulate oils, cellular debris, dust, and perspiration etc., as illustrated below. With fever, these materials seem to accumulate, more rapidly than with the average healthy (or non febrile) individual. These substances provides a media for growth of microorganisms e.g. bacteria, fungi, and can result in scalp infections with varying degrees of irritation, tenderness and in some cases---pain. This can lead to irritability---even insomnia.

For this reason, it was necessary to devise a suitable methodology for cleaning the hair and scalp; the method Dᴀʀᴀ⁺ʀ, required smaller volumes of water and can be carried out in a limited work area or space available at the bedside.

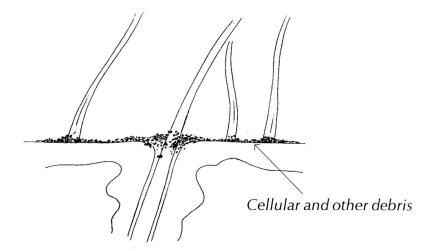

Cellular and other debris

✳ **Dara⁺r** can be performed on patients in either a supine (lying on the back and face up), where patients must remain face down, (prone position) or in a fetal position.

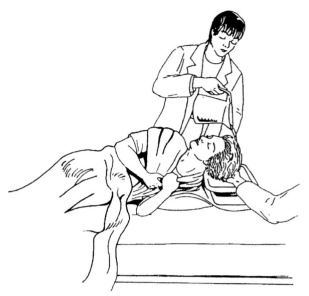

✳ **Dara⁺r** benefits people who are unable to stand too long, enter a bathtub, or a shower stall for the period of time required for traditional hairwashing.

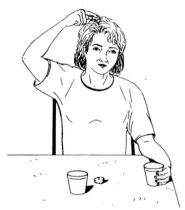

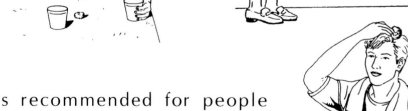

✳ **Dara⁺r** is recommended for people who use wheelchairs and for those who can wash their hair themselves.

✳· Only 2 cups (6 oz. each) of water containing a small amount of shampoo are needed for washing the hair and 2 pints of water (quart) containing a very small amount of alcohol are required for rinsing the hair.

✳· Manipulation of the scalp with a hair brush and your fingers acts to loosen, stimulate and increase the circulation of blood in the scalp and helps to promote healthier hair.

✳· Helps to relieve itchy scalps, reduce dandruff (sometime caused by eczema and/or psoriasis) and removes oily dandruff.

✳· Both patient and the bed are kept cleaner and dryer.

✳· Most brands of shampoo can be used---including those that are rinseless or waterless.

✳· **DARA⁺R**, if used on salon clients, would eliminate the hyperextension that usually occurs in salons when the head is bent backward over the sink for rinsing. With **DARA⁺R**, brushing and washing can be carried out in the salon booth then the client would be escorted to the sink, instructed to bend over the sink and rinsed as shown on page 41.

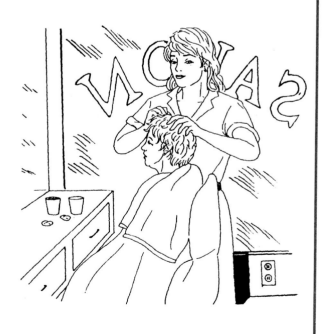

In the early eighteenth century, people learned that brushing their hair daily helped to remove dust, or loose dandruff from the hair as a way to keep the hair clean. Of course the bristles used were obtained from the boar. These natural bristle brushes did not cause problems for the users and the boar bristles were readily available. Of recent years, less expensive synthetic hair brushes (also combs) have been manufactured which, unlike boar bristles (still available), have a greater tendency to produce electrostatic charges on the hair. When these items are passed re-

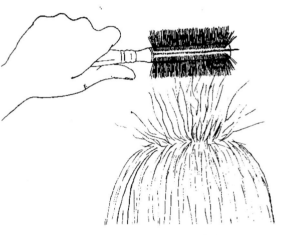

Electrostatically charged hair

peatedly through certain types of hair, the charges (on the hair) cause the hair to become unmanageable.

✳· A synthetic hair brush works well when the tips of each bristle is coated with rubber to eliminate static on the hair.

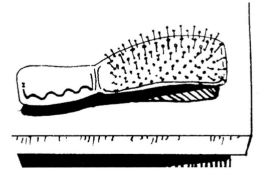

Rubber tip coated half-round hair brush

Items listed below are needed for **DARA⁺R**, many of these items, such as pillows, towels, alcohol, and wash basin, you can expect to find in any home or health care facility.

* Bed protector or large plastic trash can liner (BP)
* Boar (preferred) or rubber tipped, half-round hair brush
* Scissors
* Disposable gloves
* Hair dryer
* Several bobby pins
* Cotton puffs (large)
* Portable wash basin (WB)
* Packets of alcohol sponges
* Talcum powder
* 1 quart container

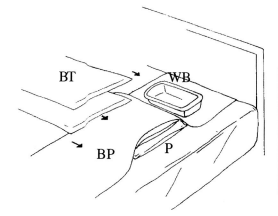

* 2 pillows (P)
* 2 bath towels (BT)
* 2 cups 6 oz. (disposable)
* 1 bottle of shampoo
* 1 bottle of (70%) isopropyl alcohol (U.S.P.)

Optional Supplies:

* 1 bottle of "leave in" hair conditioner
* Pincher clips
* Face mask (surgical)

Preperation

> **Supplies:**
> * 2- 6 oz Cups   * Cotton puffs
> * Bottle of shampoo

There are many fine shampoo products available on the market that are capable of removing oil, dirt, dandruff, odors and other undesirable substances. The chief advantage of using a good shampoo is its ability to soften---damaged, dry, and brittle hair and/or assist in correcting deep-seated dandruff.

* Most of us, through personal experience have a favorite shampoo that can be used in preparing the washing solution to be employed in DARA+R.

1. Fill a cap (from the top of a shampoo bottle) with shampoo. If the cap is large---use half a capful of shampoo. Pour the shampoo into one of the 6 ounce disposable cup and fill it with warm water.

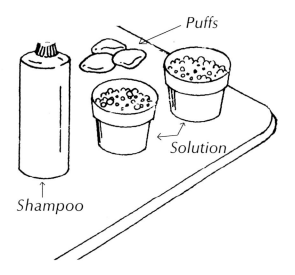

Puffs

Solution

Shampoo

2. Prepare a second cup with an equal amount of the above ingredients; place both cups containing the diluted shampoo on the patient's over bed table or tray.

Preperation

Supplies:
* Quart container   * Isopropyl alcohol

This solution is an effective rinsing formula. It consists of a small amount of isopropyl alcohol, diluted with a large amount of water, for use as a hair and scalp cleaner. The alcohol in the solution is safe since hair is basically strong and the small amount of alcohol used evaporates too quickly to be a problem e.g. adversely effecting the structure of the hair. The rinsing solution is prepared as follows:

1. Add 3 capfuls of isopropyl alcohol (70%) to a 1 quart container, as illustrated, (with a pouring spout, if available) with approximately 32 oz. of warm water. Place the container on the bedside dresser or tray next to the patient's bed.

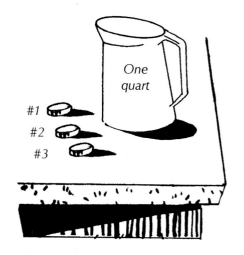

One quart

#1
#2
#3

2. Use 1/3 of a capful alcohol to a quart of water, or water alone, for the patient with an irritated scalp.

* Some manufacturer's of perm products recommend using a capful of the alcohol to a cup of water and several drops of conditioner to remove any unpleasant odor from the permed hair. The newly formed curls after a perm will not relax or loosen when this solution is used, whereas curls will relax when conventional hairwashing products e.g. shampoo, is used to wash the hair immediately after perming.

Supplies:
- ✳ Shampoo Solution
- ✳ Cotton puffs
- ✳ Hair brush
- ✳ Comb
- ✳ Hair dryer
- ✳ Rinsing Solution
- ✳ Antiseptic/alcohol sponge
- ✳ Scissors (for trim, if requested)
- ✳ Bobby pins/pincher clips
- ✳ Hair conditioner (optional)

1. Clear the over bed table or tray you intend to use; wipe table with an antiseptic solution or with an alcohol sponge; wash your hands; place supplies, as illustrated below, that you will need on the table.

2. Find a convenient electric outlet for the hair dryer (if you intend to use this device); place in the middle of the table.

3. The Rinsing Solution should be placed on the top of the bedside dresser or bureau beside the patient's bed, to prevent accidental spilling of the pitcher's contents.

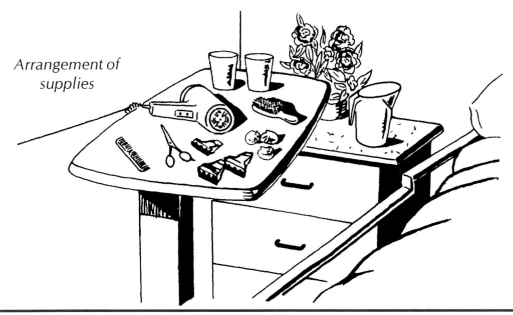

Arrangement of supplies

Supplies:
* 2 bath towels   * Wash basin
* 2 pillows   * Bed protector

1. Ask ASSISTANT to close any opened window(s), door(s), draw curtain for patient's comfort and privacy. Meanwhile, talk to the patient to establish confidence in you and briefly outline what you intend to do.

2. Have the ASSISTANT carefully raise the patient. Position two pillows (P) under patient's back and shoulders.

3. Cover pillows with bed protector (BP), extend the protector as far as possible to the "head" of the bed; place wash basin (WB) just beyond patient's head on the protector.

4. Place two towels (T) over bed protector; (if the position of the patient makes the patient uncomfortable---omit the pillow(s). Have the patient carefully lowered onto towels (Observe Warnings with bed rail).

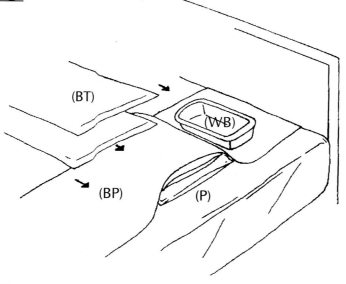

DARA⁺R METHODOLOGY

A 20 Minute Treatment

The objective of DARA⁺R Method were discussed earlier and the methodology will be described in the following pages with the appropriate illustrations. In essence, the method consists of three stages.

STAGE #1 is an initial brushing of the hair to remove any free or loose particulates e.g. debris, dust, dirt, that can be removed mechanically by proper use of a hair brush.

STAGE #2 additional contaminates such as accumulated salts (sweat), lipids (oil, greases) are removed from the hair and scalp by applying a cotton puff containing small quantities of diluted shampoo to the scalp and hair. The puffs, when held against the scalp and hair, help dissolve water soluble materials and to disperse, or suspend, insoluble substances. Other substances that physically adhere to the cotton are also removed. When the entire scalp has been treated and all of the hair is similarly treated, then water soluble, dispersed or suspended substances are absorbed with a towel. The DARA⁺R's success and effectiveness results from its unique step "R" (Rotate). The rotating of the puff increases the amount of contact, and the time, the shampoo remains on the scalp and hair. This markedly improves its cleaning effectiveness.

STAGE #3 is further cleaning obtained by rinsing the hair and scalp with a highly diluted alcohol solution, (in some cases, water alone) to remove the shampoo and any remaining contaminants.

✳· Most people, especially bedridden patients, feel refreshed when the hair and scalp is revived after washing---a feeling that only water passing over the scalp can give.

Brushing The Hair

Before proceeding with this phase of ᴅᴀʀᴀ⁺ʀ, the following precautions should be considered.

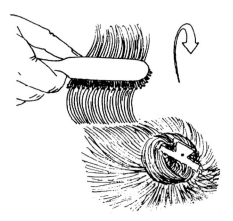

❋ <u>Omit</u> brushing the hair if the patient's head is irritated or overly sensitive.

❋ <u>Do</u> <u>not</u> brush or comb the hair to clear knots, tangles or loosen dandruff, as they will be dealt with <u>after</u> washing and <u>before</u> rinsing.

1. Slowly and <u>carefully</u> comb patient's hair; part hair in 4 separate sections; fasten each with pincher clips; do not pin hair in neck area. Place wash basin just beyond patient's head on the bed protector. Using the comb, part hair in strands 1" thick by 3" wide; hold strand upward between index and third fingers; with other hand, lay brush bristles against the scalp; rotate or turn wrist slowly while sweeping brush through this strand. Repeat 3 or 4 times; fasten sections of hair with pincher clips for convenience.

2. Use a comb to remove loose hair and debris that adheres to the brush; place hair and debris in wash basin; wipe comb and brush on a hand towel each time a strand is brushed. Continue in same manner for all of the remaining hair.

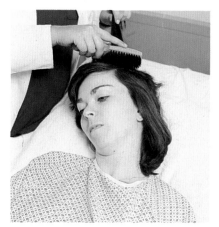

Washing The Hair And Scalp

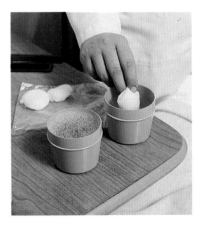

DAMPEN cotton puff by immersing it in one of the cups of washing solution; remove puff; compress between fingers so cotton will be saturated with the solution (but not dripping).

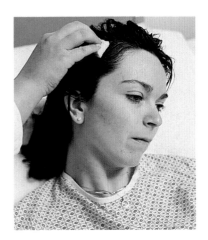

APPLY puff against the scalp and hair; press gently so that area beneath the puff will be wet with the solution---application should begin 1" to 2" behind the hairline.

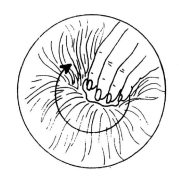

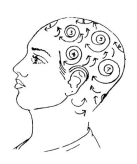

ROTATE puff to obtain active cleaning of hair and scalp;continue to **DAMPEN**, **APPLY** puff until the scalp including around the ears, neck, hairline and all hair has been treated or made wet with the cleaning solution. *THEN*

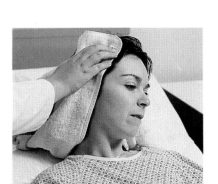

ABSORB dirty solution (before rinsing); place towel from shoulders over patients head; press gently; gather hair within the towel; squeeze gently; then gently rub the hair with the towel; keep towel around patients shoulders; discard remainder of this solution.

Repeat---→

2nd Cup (Washing Solution)

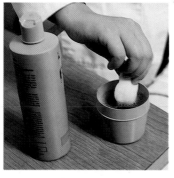 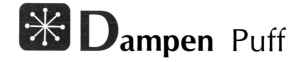

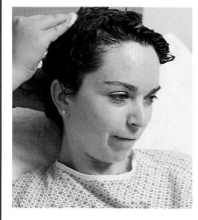

Apply to Scalp

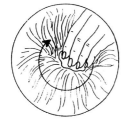

Rotate on Scalp

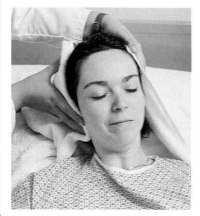

Absorb Soiled Water

Rinsing ------------------>

Treating "Tangled" Hair

1. After you tell patient you will clear the tangles from the hair; follow the product's directions for *applying* a suitable Hair Conditioner. Place one thumb of each hand below crown area and "weave" thumbs through tangled hair; place fingers of one hand over sectioned hair. Lift the separated section of hair and fasten to top of crown with pincher clip(s).

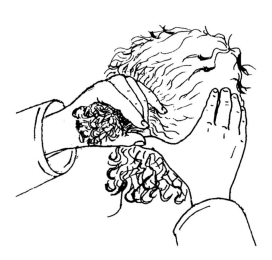

2. Lift one tangled tuft of hair in neck area; use a wide spaced tooth comb; start combing near the "ends", slowly and gently draw the comb away from the ends to loosen or clear tangles; insert the comb once again but closer to head; and comb; continue until the hair in the neck is free of tangles; then repeat for hair on the sides of the head. Release pinned section on top of crown and back of crown (crepe); repeat this step combing layer-by-layer until all of the hair is easily combed.

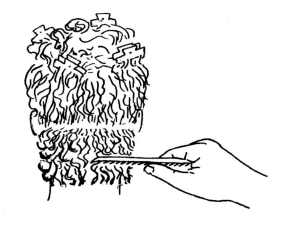

Rinsing The Hair

1. Ask ASSISTANT to lift patient high enough for you to insert 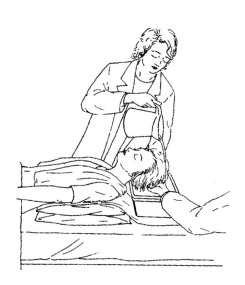 the pillow(s) under bed protector and under the patient's back. This is to have the bedridden's head beyond the pillow to expose neck area at which time the ASSISTANT supports the patient's head, and with other hand holds wash basin under patient's head--- (pausing periodically to be sure the patient is comfortable) proper alignment of the head must be maintained.

2. Maneuver your fingers (of one hand) through the hair then behind patient's neck for support of the head; and ask ASSISTANT to bend patient's ears forward so as to cover the opening of the ear while you rinse near each ear. Instruct the patient (if alert and responsive) to close their eyes while rinsing.

3. Slowly pour the Rinsing Solution with your free hand; start just beyond hairline; slowly turn the patient's head---only

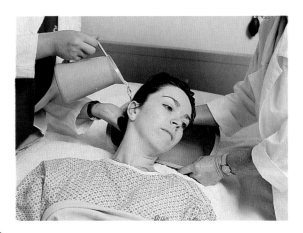
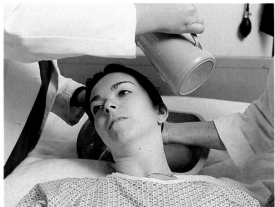

enough to expose neck area for rinsing. Continue pouring until the entire volume of Solution has been used. Gently squeeze water from the hair; ask ASSISTANT to remove towel and wash basin and place nearby.

4. Cover patient's head with the second towel (from shoulders); "towel" dry hair in neck area, ears and hairline with a gentle upward motion. Proceed with one of the recommended mini hairstyles described in the following pages (if styling is requested). If not, blow-dry the hair, (Observe Warnings with hair dryer and bed rail).

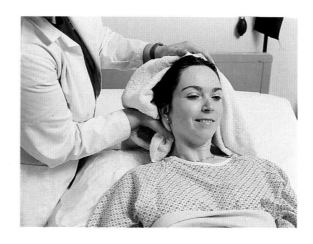

✳ For patients with long, thick hair, additional rinsing may be necessary; refill pitcher with warm water; rinse hair; place wet hair in a towel; twist towel and hair to squeeze "out" as much water as possible; ask ASSISTANT to remove towel and wash basin and place nearby.

✳ Keep bed protector in place if patient, or family has requested additional services e.g. trimming of the hair, permanent wave or mini facial.

Supplies:
* Comb
* Scissors
* Wash basin
* Pincher clips (6-8)
* Talcum powder

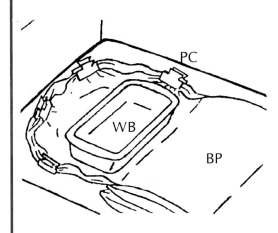

1. Usually, the bed protector (BP) is still in place after **DARA·R**, edges of protector are crimped with pincher clips (PC) to form an elevated border; center wash basin (WB) on protector just beyond patient's head (in order to contain or to catch hair during trimming); place supplies nearby and a towel around patient's neck---extended over the shoulders.

2. Comb and gently part hair into 4 sections; omit the hair in neck area, cheeks and hairline; pin hair in each section with pincher clips. Comb hair over the ears, cheek and forehead; place open scissors at desired length; close the blade to cut or trim; hold trimmed hair and place hair in wash basin for disposal. Repeat for hair on the other side of the neck; then comb the remaining hair down over the middle of the neck and trim hair to desired length.

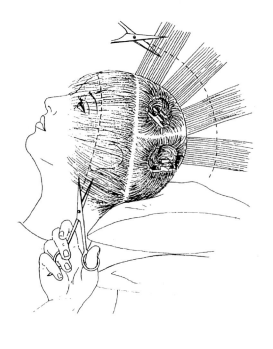

3. Remove pincher clip from a section or tuft of hair located on the back of the crown (crepe); part the hair with a comb to form a tuft of hair about 2" wide by 1/2" thick (pin remaining section of hair); 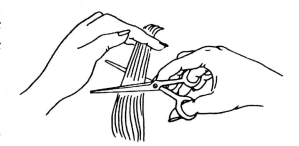 comb at right angle, or away from the scalp and hold the tuft of hair between the middle and index finger; use enough traction on the hair to keep it taut; place opened scissors over the tuft of hair at desired length and close the blade to trim; hold trimmed hair i.e. excess hair, and place this hair in wash basin for disposal; then use the length of the remaining hair in the tuft as a guide for trimming other similar tufts of hair.

4. Remove clips from the top of the crown; repeat step 3; then trim each side of the head at the desired length. Use care using scissors when trimming around patient's ears, neck and above the eyes.

5. Carefully comb hair throughout the head to remove loose hair; fold towel as you remove it from patient's shoulders; sprinkle talcum powder on the patient's skin; use the corner of the towel as a brush to remove loose hair from the patient's face and neck; roll bed protector carefully in order to contain loose hair inside of it; place nearby. Select a mini hairstyle described on the following pages, if requested. If not, blow-dry the hair in place. Observe Warnings (when using the hair dryer).

✳ The term trimming refers to lightly cutting the hair to return the hair to an already existing pattern or design lines.

TRIMMING HAIR

Out-Of-Bed

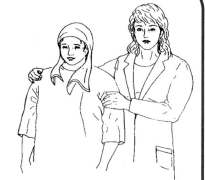

> **Supplies:**
> * Comb
> * Scissors
> * Bath towels
> * Pincher Clips
> * Plastic bag trash can liner

1. Clear the table you intend to use; place comb, scissors and clips on the table; then move table near the chair; be sure the chair used has an arm-rest; wash your hands. Cover and wrap patient's head with a clean towel; ask ASSISTANT, when the decision has been made or permission obtained, to prepare the patient to get out-of-bed and safely escort to a chair. Open top of the plastic bag; fold one side of bag over the top back edge of the chair so as to form a pocket (for collecting trimmed hair for easy disposal).

2. Gently comb hair; follow "Trimming The Hair: procedures, steps 3 to 5 on previous page or use your technique; hold trimmed hair i.e. excess hair, and place this hair in the plastic bag draped over the back of the chair. Repeat in this manner for remaining hair, (wipe any loose hair that has fallen to the floor with a moistened tissue(s).

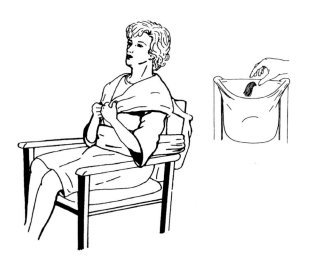

3. Carefully comb hair throughout the remainder of the head to remove any loose hair; fold towel and remove from patient's shoulders. Ask ASSISTANT to safely escort patient back into the bed. Select a mini hairstyle described on following pages, if requested. If not, blow-dry the hair in place. Observe Warnings (when using the hair dryer).

Out-Of-Bed

Supplies:
* ✳ Rinsing formula
* ✳ Cotton puffs
* ✳ Bath towel

1. Cover and wrap patient's head with a clean towel; ask AS-SISTANT when the decision has been made, or permission obtained, to prepare the patient to get out of bed and to safely escort to the sink as shown on previous page; place supplies within easy reach of the sink to be used, whether it is located in a kitchen or bathroom. Be sure patient has a piece

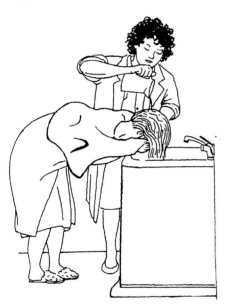

of cotton puff in each of their ears unless the patient objects; cover each eye with a corner of the towel; have the patient bend forward from the waist with her/his head over the sink and the bulk of hair falling forward i.e. over the front of the face; place one hand under the hair that draped over the front of the patient's face and use your hand to deflect the water away from the face.

2. Slowly pour the Rinsing Solution over and through patient's hair and into the sink; place thumb behind ear and bend the ears gently forward to occlude the opening to the ear while rinsing in that area; rinse thoroughly; gently squeeze excess water from hair. "Towel dry" hair, ears, neck and hairline in a gentle motion; wrap dry towel around patient's head. Ask ASSISTANT to help safely escort patient back and into the bed. Select a mini hairstyle described on following pages, if requested. If not, blow-dry the hair in place. Observe Warnings (when using the hair dryer).

CHAPTER 3

Selected Hairstyles

The three methods of styling hair of women and one for men, described on the following pages, are intended to give each patient a "finishing touch" that best suits the individual. Depending on differences in the type, the density, the length, and color of the hair, the patient's age, and also on outstanding facial characteristics, each of these factors alone, or in combination, are used to select the hairstyle that enhances the patient's appearance and provide an individual "look" that is most complimentary.

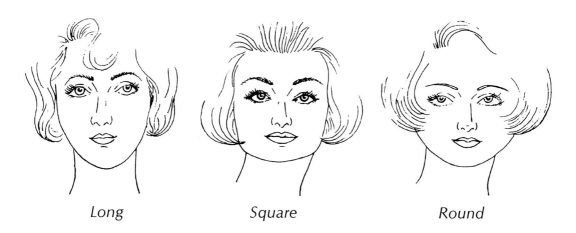

Long   Square   Round

※· These methods of altering the shape and pattern of the hair were selected because each is relatively simple to perform i.e. require less of your time, are easier on the patient (eliminates the need for rollers, and overhead hair dryer) but still provide a pleasing hair style.

※· When styling is completed, allow the bedridden access to a hand mirror to observe their hair to determine whether or not she/he is pleased with the results.

Feather The Layers

Supplies:
* Hair dryer   * Comb

1. Gently "towel dry" the hair; comb hair on one side of the head---including the temple area and behind the ears in upward sweeping movements of the comb; press hair downward over the ear; release your hand without disturbing the feather design; repeat this step for the other side of the head, then finger fluff hair on the top of crown.

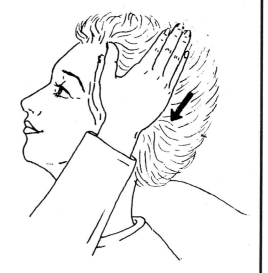

2. Set hair dryer on medium heat; with the fingers of one hand, hold the hair in the feather design on one side of the head; with other hand hold hair dryer approximately 12" away from the patients head; allow warm air from dryer to flow through your opened fingers; dry that section; repeat for other side of the head. Observe Warnings (when using the hair dryer).

3. Blow-dry the rest of the hair; comb layer-by-layer; fluff the hair as a finishing touch.

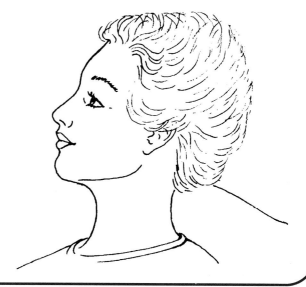

Style By Finger Rolling

> **Supplies:**
> ✳ Hair dryer   ✳ Comb
> ✳ Bobby pins

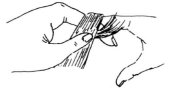

1. Start with hair that is "towel dry"; begin combing at front hairline; part and lift an average amount of tuft or hair; (do not divide hair into sections); comb tuft of hair upward and use enough traction to keep hair taut. Fold tuft over center of index finger; hold with thumb of same hand; place index finger of other hand between tuft and finger holding hair, release thumb and quickly roll the ends of tuft toward base of hair as in "twiddling"; pin securely on scalp with bobby pins on both sides of this cylindrical roll.

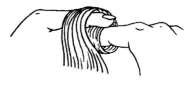

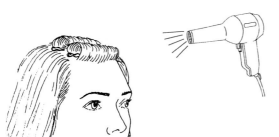

2. Repeat step 1 for additional rolls; set hair dryer on medium heat; hold approximately 12" away from the patient's head (remember—some patients do not feel pain so Be Careful) and aim dryer on rolls first. Fluff balance of hair upward with other hand while blow-drying; remove pins from rolls; Comb gently with remaining hair.

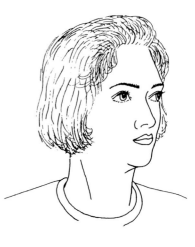

Finger Fluff

Supplies:
* Hair dryer * Comb

⁂ For patients with straight hair, styling is accomplished by using the fingers to stretch and alter the hair to render it a line e.g. slight wave, so that the hair will have greater fullness (fluff).

1. Begin directing the hair from the rear crown area of the head toward the patient's face; repeat several times until the hair adjusts to its new arrangement. Set hair dryer on medium heat; hold and direct it approximately 12" away from the patient's head.

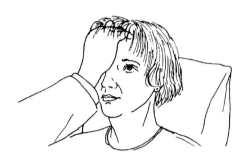

2. Spread fingers of one hand and insert fingers into the hair at hairline of the forehead; close fingers to trap the hair between the fingers. Gently withdraw the hand to provide slight traction and lift the hair; open the fingers to release the hair and allow it to fall naturally. Repeat this step throughout the top of the head; then repeat for the sides of the head in the cheek area.

3. Repeat step 2 for the remaining hair i.e. gently lifting and drying the hair. Fluff the hair with a comb as a finishing touch. <u>Observe Warnings</u> (when using the hair dryer).

"Tousle" Styling

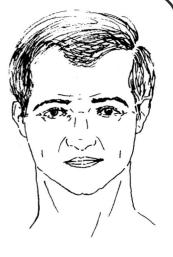

> **Supplies:**
> ✳ Comb   ✳ Hair dryer
> ✳ Scissors   ✳ Pincher clip

✳ The following technique is recommended for *thin, unruly* curly hair, a cowlick (tuft of hair which forms in a swirl effect on either side of the back part of the crown) and for a *receding hairline*---creating a more carefree look that is relatively maintenance free.

1. Gently comb patient's hair from behind the back of the head, at crown area, toward the face; repeat several times. When the hair adjusts to its new arrangement, lift the hair and part frontal area with the other hand; comb over forehead; pin the remaining hair that is in your hand; then section hair below receding area and pin, as illustrated.

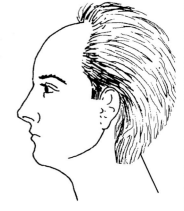

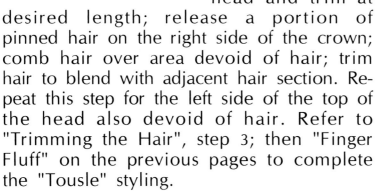

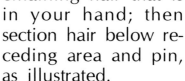

2. Place scissors over the hair in the middle of forehead and trim at desired length; release a portion of pinned hair on the right side of the crown; comb hair over area devoid of hair; trim hair to blend with adjacent hair section. Repeat this step for the left side of the top of the head also devoid of hair. Refer to "Trimming the Hair", step 3; then "Finger Fluff" on the previous pages to complete the "Tousle" styling.

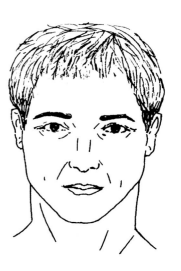

CHAPTER 4

Other Cosmetology Specialties

In the previous chapters, your focus has been on background: what goes into preparing the patient, the over bed table and/or tray, and how to perform a number of different CosmeCare procedures e.g. washing, trimming and styling the patients hair. In this chapter methodology has been expanded to include other cosmetology specialties and will include, the mini-facial, manicure and pedicure.

The mini-facial service involves the treatment of the skin to maintain or improve the health of the skin by cleaning, increasing circulation and correcting excessive dryness or oiliness of the skin. While partial permanent waving and haircoloring may seem to be time consuming, understanding the nature of these procedures beforehand and the benefits to the patient can be rewarding in obtaining successful results. Care of a wig or hairpiece is reasonably easy to provide or perform. Procedure for manicures and pedicures are provided along with discussions of potential problems that may arise when services are rendered to patients. Shaving or trimming of a beard and mustache may be more challenging. Most men before being bedridden developed, or established, over time, a methodology that gives results they feel is most pleasing to him. The patient may have their own favorites i.e. want to use their own supplies and/or equipment such as hand lotion, skin cream, haircolor, or a particular comb attachment to use with the electric clipper.

✳ Before proceeding with the service involving the face and nails, a discussion of some of the lesions that occur on the face is in order.

Lesions Of The Face

Earlier in the book, attempts were made to describe some of the lesions you might encounter on the scalp and nails when providing CosmeCare to the patient. When providing services e.g. facials, in all likelihood face lesion(s) would be recognized and appropriate action would be taken by trained medical professionals for patients in health care facilities, or by the patient themselves or family member(s), if at home.

In addition to lesions listed (with precautions) that were given earlier for patients with local and systemic infectious diseases, the list of possible lesions observed on the face is undoubtedly considerably longer than for the scalp (where the hair affords some protection to underlying skin) in view of the following factors:

✳ Greater exposure to direct sunlight (ultraviolet radiation)

✳ Greater contact whether from the same, or among different individuals, e.g. from hand to face, face to face, lip to face, etc.

✳ Lesions from mechanical trauma e.g. scratching (or squeezing) following irritation from insect bites, blackheads, or pimples, etc.

✳ Allergic reaction, manifested and easily visible, in the skin of the face from food, medication, perfumes, and/or cosmetics.

✳ Higher chance of contact dermatitis from greater use of topically applied cosmetics of markedly different chemical composition and consistency.

PIGMENTATION - Lesions with pigmentation abnormalities, induced locally or systemically by use of drugs/medication, diseases, trauma, hormonal imbalance. For example, in vitiligo the pigment cells (melanocytes) are destroyed and a spot or area will be much lighter (or have no color) than the surrounding skin.

VIRAL LESIONS - Although viral lesions of the face were mentioned and discussed earlier, two viral infections are worthy of note.

a). *Cold Sores* (Herpes Simplex) is an acute, often recurrent viral infection and seems to be provoked by many factors e.g. fever, sunburn, nervousness, fatigue, trauma. The lesion consists of small groups of vesicles on a base of swollen tissue especially around the mouth.

b). *Shingles* (Herpes Zoster) this is an acute lesion that results in severe pain along a nerve followed by a group of vesicles on one side of the face (although the infection can occur elsewhere). Most patients recover without any residual effects, but some show some pain for months or years and/or some facial paralysis. Most adults are familiar with cold sores; less so with shingles. These are both contagious and are thought to be the same virus as that causing "chicken pox". There is evidence that the risk of transmitting the virus is a short time before and short time after the final lesions have crusted, although most adults have already been exposed to this virus.

✳ <u>Suggested</u> <u>Course</u> <u>of</u> <u>Action</u>: If these lesions are present when you arrive at the bedside; delay any procedure until you speak to the patient's ASSIGNED NURSE. If there is no pain and the lesions are almost healed, permission will probably be given.

TUMORS - These lesions when present on the patient's face are in plain view of health professionals in charge of the patient in health facilities, in-home and hospice care. There is little likelihood that the skin tumors listed below would be overlooked. Still, if a mass is observed, it should be noted and reported to the ASSIGNED NURSE.

a). *Malignant melanoma* - This tumor is responsible for most of the deaths caused by skin cancer. The tumors vary in color, from flesh tints to black---and frequently blue, purple, red.

b). *Squamous cell carcinoma* - This tumor occurs most often on exposed area of fair skinned individuals who tan poorly.

c). *Basal cell carcinoma* - A slow growing tumor found most often on exposed areas.

✳ Suggested Course of Action: If permission is given for a mini facial, then it (facial) could be provided for those with squamous and basal carcinoma. The Malignant melanoma is highly invasive and the survival is relatively short after the tumor spreads from the original site. Once the tumor has already spread a facial could be given---would you want to if it made the patient feel better?

Supplies:

* Face cream
* Face pack
* Facial tissues
* Cotton puffs
* Skin freshener
* Cleansing cream
* Antiseptic/alcohol sponge
* Hand/bath towels

1. Clear the table you intend to use; wipe table with anti-septic solution or with an alcohol sponge; place supplies on the table; wash your hands. Refer to "Patient Preparation" Chapter 2; ask an ASSISTANT to move and position the patient for comfort toward the "foot" of the bed, if possible; cover patient's hair, clothing and bedspread with clean towels; keep neck uncovered; cover each patient's eyes with a damp (not wet) cotton puff. You should sit at the "head" of the bed for easy access to the patient and supplies.

2. Remove cover of cleanser cream jar; use a facial tissue to remove a half to one teaspoon from the jar; apply cream to patient's neck and bring the cream up and onto the face using upward movements, and spread cream over the entire face; wait a few minutes; remove cream containing residues e.g. dust, oils, exfoliated cells with clean facial tissue(s).

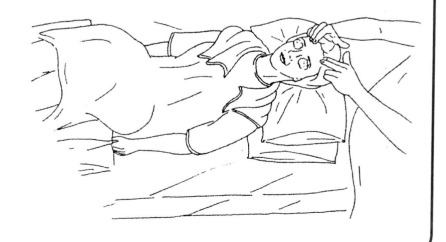

3. Apply chosen face pack to the skin; follow product's direction as to *mixing, application, duration and removal* of this material from the skin; then gently pat skin freshener to the skin with a cotton puff.

4. Remove from the face cream container an amount of cream equal to approximately one or two teaspoons with a facial tissue and apply to the face using an upward motion; then apply over the patient's neck, chin, around the mouth, cheeks, while stroking and massaging the skin in a slow rhythmic manner----finishing at the forehead. Remove towel from patient's head; prepare for ᴅARA⁺R (Chapter 2) if hairwashing is requested.

✳ After the facial is completed you may be requested to apply one or more of the bedridden's favorite cosmetics.

Every one of us should be familiar with normal appearing nails, in as much as we have 10 on the hands, 10 on the toes and years of personal experience observing them. Based on this background, it follows that if you are providing nail care for a patient, you should be able to recognize abnormal changes in the nail or adjacent tissues—even if you are unable to identify the cause or nature of the abnormality.

It might be helpful to review briefly the anatomy of the nail, keeping in mind that nails, like hair, are appendages of the skin. They arise from epidermal cells that are similar in structure to cells in ordinary skin, except that the cells in the nails become converted to keratin, as convex laminated sheets i.e. nail plate.

STRUCTURE

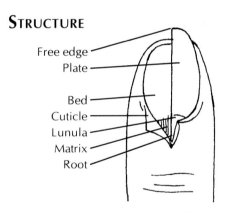
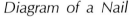

Diagram of a Nail

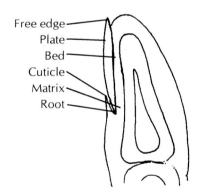

Cross Section of a Nail

The nail bed is very similar to corium layer of cells in plain skin. New growth of nail occurs at the base of the nail (or root) in a group of cells that make up the matrix. The nail is firmly attached to the cuticle. As new cells are formed on the nail plate, the nail increases in length and moves outward. The lunula, located near the root, is a small crescent shaped whitish area (since it has fewer blood vessels, and a less transparent nail plate).

NAIL DISORDERS

Disorders of the nail structure, whether from local or systemic origins, may be manifested by the nail becoming so brittle that they can fray, split or even separate. The nail can show depressions, wavy ridges, spots, indentations, thin nail plates (eggshell nail). Blue colored nails can be due to poorly oxygenated blood (e.g. in disorders of the heart) or inadequate blood circulation.

Most patients with a nail disorder may receive a manicure or pedicure (with care), if the nail or adjacent tissue is <u>not</u> involved in an infective process. If you are unsure, you should consider having the patient obtain a medical opinion before giving a manicure or pedicure or even covering the nails with a nail polish---*especially* if there is redness, swelling, soreness and discomfort when the nail is touched.

Nail abnormalities can result from local insults e.g. infection, by physical trauma and exposure to chemicals such as agents used in industry, the home, (occasionally in the salon). In the latter, alteration in nails and adjacent tissues can be induced in some individuals by contact with detergent soaps, use of nail polish, nail polish remover and/or application of fake (acrylic) nails. Changes in nail structure, color, and growth are frequently manifestations of abnormalities in body function or disease. These include thyroid gland dysfunction, rheumatoid arthritis, psoriasis, drug reactions, anemia, allergies, radiation (x-rays), as well as systemic infections from a large variety of pathogenic microorganisms or germs.

HANG-NAILS - This abnormally occurs when a piece of the skin or cuticle at the base of nail becomes detached. The importance of hang-nails is the infection that can result. The organism involved are usually bacteria or molds that enter through the break in the skin of the hang-nail. The infection may follow around the edge of the nail and extend beneath the nail resulting in swelling, pain, and/or purulent (pus) pockets.

✳· Suggested Course of Action - If any redness, swelling, tenderness, or any other signs of inflammation are observed, the ASSIGNED NURSE should be notified and nail care delayed until permission is granted. In most instances, in the absence of infection, nail care may be carried out if the nail involved i.e. hang-nail is treated with an antiseptic before anything is done.

IN-GROWN NAIL - This condition usually results from improper trimming of the nail (usually the toe) by filing (or cutting) the nail too deeply in the corners. Improperly fitting shoes, stubbing a toe and failing to correct hangnails are also given as contribution factors for in-grown nails. When the tissue around the involved nail becomes red, swollen, painful etc., it usually indicates existence of an infection and inflammation.

✳· Suggested Course of Action - It is best to report this condition to the ASSIGNED NURSE. As soon as the nail(s) problem is corrected and the nail is growing normally, apply a suitable cream or lotion to the nails to soften cuticles before carrying out any nail procedure.

RINGWORM OF THE NAILS, HANDS AND FEET (Athletes Foot) - Ringworm is a disease used to describe several species of fungi that only infects the skin, hair and nails. The infection can be deeply seated and give rise to colorless vesicles (blisters) on the skin of the hands and feet. Under conditions that favor the growth of this organism, the infection can spread to other un-infected areas in the same individual and to others not previously infected.

RINGWORM OF THE NAILS (Tinea Unguium) The fungus grows on the nail surface and can involve deeper layers of the nail plate. Infections of the toenails are more common than that of fingernails. The infected nails become thickened and lusterless and cellular debris tend to accumulate under the free edge of the nail. The nail plate can become separated. These infections are sometimes difficult to eradicate and may persist and flare up on occasions over many years.

✳. <u>Suggested</u> <u>Course</u> <u>of</u> <u>Action</u> - Patients with these infections should be reported to the **ASSIGNED NURSE** in order to identify the organism and initiate treatment with prescriptions for antifungal medication, that include oral dosage forms as well as topical medications. As soon as the infection has been adequately treated, or cleared, a pedicure can be initiated. Antifungal powders, liquid and ointment are available to prevent ringworm reinfection, and are the method of choice. It is essential to keep the affected area <u>dry</u> and cool.

Supplies:
* Emery boards
* Cotton puffs
* Hand towel
* Nail remover (acetone)
* Antiseptic/alcohol sponge

Commercially available are artificial nail removal products. Commonly used products consist of a jar, that usually contains either soft brushes or sponge, with a chemical ingredients e.g. acetone, to safely and easily remove the artificial nails, nail tips, and any residual glue---without damaging the natural nails.

1. Clear the table you intend to use; wipe table with an antiseptic or with an alcohol sponge; wash your hands. Refer to "Patient Preparation" Chapter 2. Cover an area on the table with a towel; then other supplies nearby; place the artificial nail remover container close to the patient's hand. Follow the directions on the product label for applying the *chemical* agent (usually a liquid solvent) to the nail, 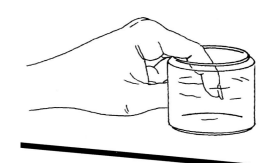 and/or *amount* of time needed for the solvent to soften the artificial nail, and the suggested method for *removing* the artificial nail. Complete the "Mini Manicure" procedure on the following page if this service is requested. <u>Do not cut the patient's cuticles.</u>

Supplies:

* ❊ Emery board
* ❊ Wash basin
* ❊ Hand/bath towels
* ❊ Cotton puffs
* ❊ Hand lotion/cream
* ❊ Orangewood stick
* ❊ Antiseptic/alcohol sponge

1. Clear the table you intend to use; wipe table with antiseptic or with an alcohol sponge; place supplies on the table; wash your hands. Refer to "Patient Preparation" Chapter 2. Fill wash basin to 1/4 of its volume with warm water; place basin on table; then adjust the table over the patient who is in bed; remove old nail polish if present.

2. Place patient's hand (left) in the warm water---place a rolled towel under the arm to support the arm for patient's comfort. Take hold of the patient's other hand (right); hold the little finger between your thumb and first two fingers; tilt emery board; file underneath the free edge of nail; beginning with one side, file toward the center; then file toward center for other side of the finger; when finished, place this hand in the wash basin with warm water.

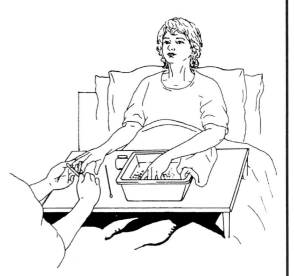

3. Remove the left hand from water and dry with a towel; file nails as noted in step 2; apply lotion or cream to the cuticles with a facial tissue; push cuticles gently with orangewood stick to loosen skin surrounding nails; do not press base of nails (matrix); clean any matter beneath free-edge of the nail with orangewood stick; reapply cream and massage the hand; gently buff nails with a cotton puff. Repeat for the right hand.

Supplies:

- ✳ 2 towels
- ✳ Emery board
- ✳ Cotton puffs
- ✳ Talcum powder
- ✳ Facial Tissues
- ✳ Wash basin
- ✳ Orangewood stick
- ✳ Foot lotion/cream
- ✳ Bottle of polish remover
- ✳ Antiseptic/alcohol sponge

1. Clear the table you intend to use; wipe table with antiseptic solution or with an alcohol sponge; place supplies on the table; wash your hands. Refer to "Patient Preparation" Chapter 2. Add to a wash basin filled with 2 inches of warm water, a small amount of mild detergent e.g. shampoo.

2. Ask ASSISTANT to position the patient so that one foot (left) can be placed in the wash basin while the patient is in bed (this will depend on whether the patient will tolerate the movement involved); apply a small amount of polish remover to a cotton puff and remove old nail polish if present.

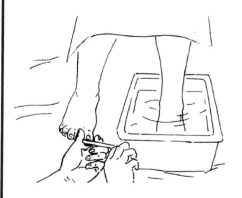

3. Hold patient's other foot (right); place small toe between your thumb and first two fingers; tilt emery board; slowly and gently file nail straight across; when finished, place this foot in the water.

4. Remove the foot (left) that was soaking from the water and wipe it dry with a towel; file nails as noted in step 2; apply foot lotion or cream on the cuticles with a facial tissue; massage the foot and remove any loose tissue surrounding cuticles with the orangewood stick; do not press at base of nails (matrix). Clean any matter that accumulated beneath the free-edge of the

nail with the orangewood stick; continue application of lotion/cream all over the foot and slowly massage area---including the ankle; gently buff nails with a cotton puff.

5. Remove the right foot from the water; remove wash basin from the bed and place nearby; continue procedure provided in step 3; sprinkle talcum powder from its container over the patient's feet and between the toes.

✳ In cases where the patient must remain supine (horizontal) and the foot cannot be placed in, or the leg rotated enough to immerse the foot in a wash basin, the soaking of the foot can be accomplished by placing the wash basin with the prepared warm water solution under the foot, soaking a towel with 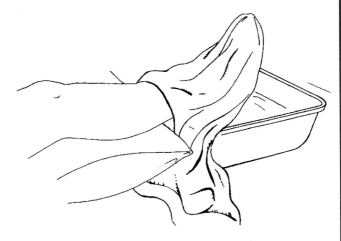 this water and wrapping it around the foot allowing it to remain for approximately 3-4 minutes; ask a qualified ASSISTANT to position patient's foot over wash basin, and support with a pillow(s). Remove towel; immerse it in the water and reapply for another 3-4 minute. The other parts of the Pedicure procedure in steps 2 to 5 are essentially comparable---then repeat for the patient's other foot.

✳ Commercially available are products to assist in removing thickened exfoliated or dead cells from the feet and ankles, elbows and knees. They are formulated to contain an abrasive to remove the layers of hard dried skin (can reduce callouses). This results in a "new" skin which is esthetically pleasing to the bedridden.

Before Using Haircolor Products

Haircolor products contain chemical agents (dyes) that have been known to produce allergic reactions in sensitized or rashes in hypersensitive individuals, e.g. itching, redness and swelling of the skin in direct contact with the material or in severe cases of allergic responses rashes occur in other, untreated, or exposed parts of the body.

Haircoloring products are manufactured and sold under regulations set forth by the Food, Drug and Cosmetic Act. It requires those who use the products, including salon professionals, to carry out preliminary skin testing before it is employed to establish that it is "safe" to use. Though a person may never have been sensitive to hair products, the responsiveness of the individual can change i.e. become sensitized. The patch or skin test takes a few minutes to perform and can be given to the patient at the time of other CosmeCare services such as a mini facial, manicure and/or pedicure. The test, however, must be carried out 48 hours before each haircolor application. Before proceeding with the patch testing of the skin, it is advisable for you to examine the hair and scalp for evident of infection and/or other lesions.

✳ A salon professional is best qualified to test the patient to ascertain whether the individual is sensitive (or allergic) to a haircolor product.

HAIRCOLORING

Supplies:
- ✳ Haircolor kit
- ✳ Latex gloves
- ✳ Wash basin
- ✳ Cotton Puffs
- ✳ Comb
- ✳ Applicator bottle
- ✳ 2 bath towels
- ✳ Plastic apron
- ✳ Antiseptic/alcohol sponge
- ✳ Empty plastic gallon container

✳ Was hypersensitivity/allergic testing performed? If yes, proceed with haircoloring if the results were *negative*---it is not necessary to wash the hair.

1. Clear the table you intend to use; wipe table with an antiseptic solution or an alcohol sponge; place supplies on the table and refer to "Patient Preparation" Chapter 2. Fill the gallon container with warm water; place on bedside dresser.

2. Prepare haircolor according to label on product; follow product's direction for *mixing* and *timing*; place bottle with haircoloring product on the table; you should wear protective gloves and apron. Cover patient's shoulders and bedspread with towel(s); place small piece of cotton puff in patient's ears.

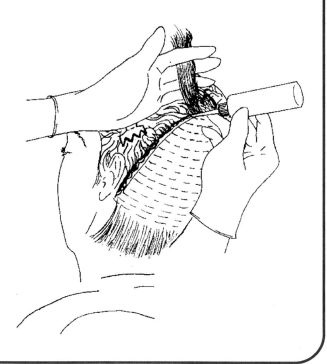

3. Gently comb hair; section hair into 4 quarters and pin

out-of-way; apply or outline partings with haircolor, release one section; use comb or squeeze bottle nozzle tip to part hair in strands or tufts 2" or 3" wide by 1/2" thick; apply haircolor. Continue this step with remaining hair and try not to touch the ends of hair with color. Allow mixture to remain on the hair for the required time and for the color to develop properly; wipe around patient's hairline, ears and neck if they become wet with haircolor.

4. Rinse haircolor using the gallon of warm water; ask an ASSISTANT to raise and support the patient's head---Refer to DARA+R (Chapter 2) for washing the hair. Remove stains from around the hairline, ears and neck; remove towel from patient's shoulders; discard haircolor mixture when cleaning. Select mini hairstyle described on previous pages, if requested. If not, blow dry the hair. <u>Observe Warnings</u> (with use of hair dryer and bed rail).

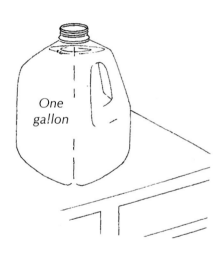

One
gallon

✳· For the patient who prefers and is able to get out-of-bed to have their hair rinsed, refer to page 41.

✳· Highlighting the hair (bleaching) require both experience and time---salon professionals are best qualified to provide this service, if requested.

PARTIAL PERMANENT WAVE

> **Supplies:**
> * Perm kit
> * Comb
> * Scissors
> * Towels
> * End wraps
> * Perm rods (assorted sizes 18-20)
> * Cotton puffs
> * Collecting vessel (pail)
> * Antiseptic/alcohol sponge
> * Empty plastic gallon container

Giving a full perm to a patient is usually not effective in terms of the time required. For this reason a partial permanent wave is recommended. To this end, the curls are formed with hair on the top and back of the crown and/or the sides, top of the crown and in the neck area.

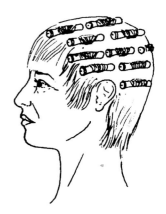

For best results, after referring to "Trimming The Hair" Chapter 3, "ends" of the hair adjacent to the area to be curled should be trimmed after perm rods are removed so that they blend with the curls that are permed. The list of different perm kits available commercially to professionals and nonprofessionals is extensive. The following information is useful before starting:

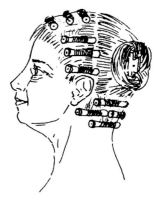

* In general, hair is washed, pretreated with conditioner if the hair is highly porous or fragile and then rinsed
* The hair is sectioned into blocks, the hair to be curled is paper wrapped on to perming rods and kept moist (water wrapped)
* A waving lotion is applied to hair on each wrapped permed rods
* Hair (and rods) are often covered with a plastic cap, the wav-

ing lotion allowed to remain for the required time and then rinsed

✳ The curled hair on each of the permed rods is treated with a neutralizer for a prescribed period of time and then rinsed

1. Clear the table you intend to use including the bedside dresser; wipe both with antiseptic solution or with an alcohol sponge; wash your hands. Refer "Patient Preparation"; use "ᗡARA⁺R" without brushing the hair (Stage #1); then follow "Trimming the Hair", if requested (or use your technique). Fill gallon container with warm water; place both gallon and quart pitcher containing Rinsing Solution on patient's bedside dresser; position collecting vessel (pail) on the floor, nearby.

✳ Follow closely directions of the Perm kit to be used for; *Precautions, Wrapping of hair, Applying waving lotion, Timing and Rinsing.*

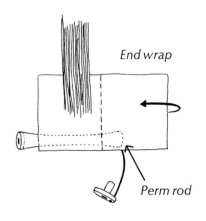

End wrap

Perm rod

2. Before processing time is completed, request an ASSISTANT to position patient and to hold and support the patient's head. At the end of the processing time, rinse hair with the gallon of warm water; make sure each curl is properly rinsed; ask the ASSISTANT to stay with the patient while you empty wash basin of the water into a sink or collecting vessel; then refill the container with additional clean warm water; rinse the hair again.

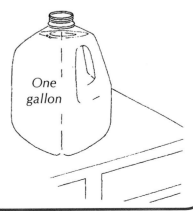

One gallon

✳ Rinse a third time if the patient's hair is excessively thick and/or long.

✳ Follow directions on the perm kit for; *Neutralizing, Timing, Removal of Perm Rods.*

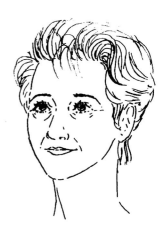

3. When finished, ask ASSISTANT to stay with patient while you fill the gallon container with warm water and a Rinsing Solution as a "final rinse"; gently rinse the hair with gallon of water; then rinse the hair with prepared Rinsing Solution in the quart pitcher, to remove perm odor and refresh the hair.

4. After rinsing; cover patient's head with a clean towel and blot the hair to remove as much water as possible, dry the ears and neck with a gentle upward motion. Select mini hairstyle described on previous pages, if styling is requested. If not, comb and blow-dry the hair, <u>Observe Warning</u> (with use of hair dryer and bed rail).

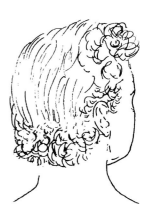

✳ For the patient who prefers and is able to get out-of-bed to have their hair rinsed, refer to page 41.

Supplies:
* Shaving cream
* Paper towels
* Wash basin
* Disposable cup
* After shave powder or lotion
* Towels (bath & hand)
* Antiseptic/alcohol sponge
* Disposable razor

1. Clean the table you intend to use; wipe table with antiseptic or alcohol sponge; Place supplies on table; fill the wash basin and disposable cup with warm water and place them on the table. Spread the bath towel around patient's neck and shoulders, wash your hands.

2. Soak hand towel in wash basin; twist towel to squeeze out water and place over the patient's face and chin; allow it to remain a few minutes (to soften the hair); remove the towel and apply a small volume (1 oz.) of shaving cream to the bearded area of the face and allow it also to remain for several minutes.

3. Hold razor at about 45 degree angle to the skin; use gentle but firm slow strokes in the direction that the hair is growing; use traction on the skin to hold the skin taut around creases. Rinse razor in cup of warm water; continue until the face is "clean". Never allow razor to move laterally (sideways) as this movement can result in cuts. To obtain a closer shave the razor should be moved against the direction of hair growth (upward).

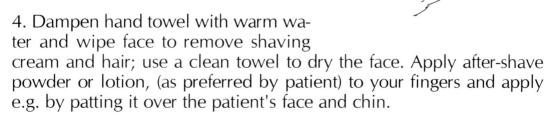

4. Dampen hand towel with warm water and wipe face to remove shaving cream and hair; use a clean towel to dry the face. Apply after-shave powder or lotion, (as preferred by patient) to your fingers and apply e.g. by patting it over the patient's face and chin.

TRIMMING A BEARD

> **Supplies:**
> * Comb
> * Scissors
> * Bath towel
> * Electric hair clipper
> * Comb attachments
> * Antiseptic/alcohol sponge

1. Clear the table you intend to use; wipe table with an antiseptic solution or with an alcohol sponge; place supplies on the table; wash your hands. Refer "Patient Preparation" Chapter 2. The patient usually knows the length of hair he prefers left on his beard and sometimes will indicate the size of comb attachment to be used on the hair clipper.

2. Cover patient's clothing and bedspread with a clean towel. Place comb attachment on clipper; begin under patient's chin; bring or move clipper (previously disinfected) upward; repeat trimming hair in rows i.e. width of clipper blade, using an upward movement. Remove comb attachment and position clipper downward; begin on one side of the neck 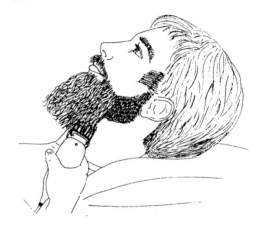 and make a definite line at the chin bone ending on the other side of the chin; continue to remove remaining hair on the neck and under the ears. Trim sideburns and beard to blend into a defined line and shape. Fold towel to enclose the trimmed hair as you remove it from patient's shoulders.

3. When possible, allow the patient access to a hand mirror in order for him to determine whether, or not, he is satisfied with the results; also, you should stand in front of the patient and look directly at his beard to be sure that the trimmed area had the desired shape and is symmetrical (with reference with the face and lips).

Supplies:
* ✳ Comb
* ✳ Scissors
* ✳ Electric hair clipper
* ✳ Face Mask (surgical)

THE MUSTACHE

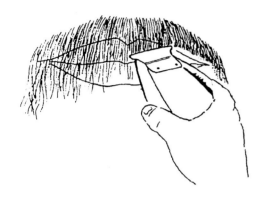

1. Prepare patient following Step #1 from the previous page "Trimming A Beard". Comb the hair of the whiskers above the mouth down over the patient's lip; hold clipper using 1 quarter of the cutting blade for trimming; start shaping whiskers from either outside corner of the lip and ending on the other side of the lip or corner. Define a clear line by trimming directly at the lip line, or according to patient's preference. Follow Step 3 from previous page, "Trimming A Beard" as a finishing procedure.

THE EYEBROWS

1. Insert the comb at the base of the hair on one eyebrow; comb the hair upward until the hair below the comb is at the desired length; hold the comb in place and with other hand, trim the longer hair i.e. hair extending beyond the top of the comb. Repeat procedure for other eyebrow.

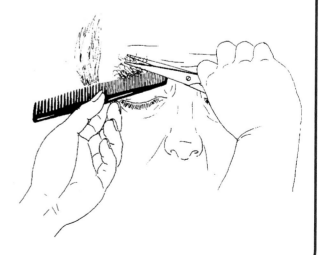

CLEANING WIGS AND HAIRPIECES

Supplies:
* Shampoo
* Towels
* Hair dryer
* Wash basin/sink
* Wig form/water pitcher

* If requested, wash whatever existing hair the patient has, vis-a-vis "Dara⁺r", "Patient Preparation" Chapter 2. Instructions on care of the wig or hairpiece are usually given on labels fixed to the inside of these items, along with information as to type of hair used e.g. human or synthetic.

* Salon professionals are best qualified to service wig(s) or hairpiece(s) made with human hair---considering the high purchase price for some of these items.

1. Immerse wig or hairpiece in a sink, or wash basin, containing at least 4 inches of warm water; and add 2 or 3 capfuls of mild shampoo (even Woolite); move the item back and forth in the solution; lift the item and allow it to drain; repeat the immersing and draining process several more times.

2. Rinse item thoroughly by filling the sink (or wash basin) with clean water; repeat the immersing and removal of the item from the water until the item is clean; hold item and allow it to drain; cover item with a dry towel and press it between your hands to facilitate removal of excess water; blow-dry or allow to air dry; place the item over a wig form (or overturned water pitcher); comb and fluff the wig or hairpiece to obtain the designed lines or style.

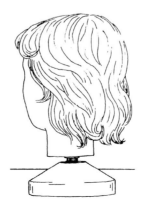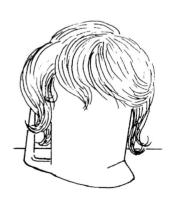

"What Is Hospice"

Hospice is a National Program that focuses on emphasizing quality health care in the final phases of a terminally ill person. It encourages the involvement of families and friends in giving care to make the dying more comfortable. Hospice patients are cared for by a team of physicians, nurses, social workers, counselors, the clergy and volunteers. The team members work closely to attend to the patient's needs and to treat the FAMILY as a "unit of care". Also, the Hospice goal is to be sure that the environment where patients and their families have satisfactory mental and spiritual preparation for the impending death. Most terminally ill persons prefer to spend their remaining time in a familiar setting e.g. their home and/ or with their family, rather than in a sterile impersonal surroundings. When a patient suffers escalating pain or other symptoms which cannot be treated at home, some hospitals have inpatient units that offer Hospice care. The patient's personal physician usually refers the terminally ill person to a local Hospice for care. The Hospice Care Team serves patients regardless of:

✳ Age, gender, race, creed
✳ Nationality, sexual orientation, disability
✳ Diagnosis, or ability to pay

Listed below are some of the selections available from the National Hospice Organization that will be of value to both the patient and you. Two of the brochures available include the following:

✳ "What's Hospice" - This brochure contains 20 Common Questions About Hospice and the hospice philosophy.

✳ "Basics of Hospice" - This brochure outlines the basics of Hospice---its philosophy, how it works, how it differs from traditional care.

To learn about Hospice in your community, check your local telephone directory or you can write and request brochures from:

The National Hospice Organization
1901 North Moore Street, Suite 901
Arlington, Virginia 22209

Call the National Hospice Helpline at: 1-800-658-8898

In addition, you can obtain information on Hospice from The American Cancer Society, The American Association of Retired Persons and the Social Security Administration.

Patients With HIV And Those With AIDS

In as much as there are thousands of people that have Human Immunodeficiency Virus (HIV) and are unaware of it, it is impossible for you to know which of your bedridden patients have been exposed and carry the HIV virus. This situation is not any different than that which exists every day in salons and where there is personal contact in performing electrolysis, esthetics, and health related services etc.

Overwhelming evidence clearly shows that the virus is transmitted via body fluids, usually HIV contaminated blood and semen and medications derived from contaminated blood and injected into patients. Similarly, casual and ordinary contact with people infected with HIV has not been shown to result in the transmission of this virus to others. In any case it pays to be careful.

When, or even if, called upon to deliver CosmeCare services to a bedridden patient in the early stages of AIDS, the requirements for transmission of the HIV virus is probably similar to that mentioned above. Each CosmeCaregiver should decide whether, or not, to respond to request for your services and the extent to which you feel comfortable with the various measures available to ensure safety e.g. gloves, mask, gowns, especially in cases of full blown AIDS. However, in view of impaired immune system that exists in these patients, it is reasonable to expect that requirements set forth by medical professionals will require sterile gowns, surgical masks, and gloves to protect the patient from microorganisms that pose little risk to you but may be pathogenic to AIDS patient.

Sanitation and Hygiene

I would be remiss not to include a brief discussion of Sanitation and Hygiene in as much as it impacts both of you, i.e. the bedridden and the CosmeCaregiver. Unfortunately, the ideal situation, asepsis (the absence of all viaible living microorganisms) is difficult or impossible to achieve in most instances. Maintaining asepsis to the extent possible benefits both the bedridden and the CosmeCaregiver. While you cannot control all sources of environmental airborne microorganisms, you can control to some extent disemination of airborne organisms i.e. between you and the bedridden by using a face mask. Control of non-airborne microorganisms can be accomplished by use of sterile surgical gloves, sterile clothing, sterile combs, scissors, etc. Obviously, although this level of asepsis is most desirable such as in a hospital operating room, it is impractical and other methods have and continue to be developed. Many of the agents used to kill or inhibit growth of non-airborne microorganisms pose health problems themselves. Such problems must be considered and are dealt with continuously by segments of the medical profession for certain instruments that cannot be autoclaved (high pressure steam). Varying degrees of asepsis can be achieved by (1) chemical agents e.g. disinfectants, antiseptics, antibiotics, gas and vapors (2) Physical agents e.g. dry and moist heat, radiation such as X-Ray and Ultraviolet, mechanical filtration (less than 0.2 micron pore sizes). Of these two groups---ultraviolet and antiseptic/disinfectants* are the ones that have been generally adapted by many in the salon industry.

The term disinfectant and antiseptic are usually used synonymously but they are different. Disinfectants are substances that are often toxic and are able to kill microorganisms, including pathogens on inanimate objects, but not spores. On the other hand, antiseptics are less toxic, less effective in killing the organism, but can be used safely to wipe the skin to destroy or prevent growth of most common disease producing microorganisms.

Throughout this book when an antiseptic was mentioned it was Isopropyl Alcohol (70%). It can kill 90% of normal bacteria found on the skin in about 2 minutes. Other chemical agents that have been used as antiseptic (or disinfectants) are detergents benzalkonium chloride 1:10,000 to 1:2,000; sodium hypochlorite (bleach) 1%, glutaraldelyde 2% in alcohol, polyvinyl pyrolidone iodine (Betadine) 2% and hydrogen peroxide 3%. Only a few of perhaps hundreds of chemical agents available and used for dis-infection have been mentioned.

In selecting the chemical agents most suitable to your needs, be-sides cost, consideration must be given to time required to achieve the desired result (inhibiting or killing), physical and chemical compatibility (or incompatibility); preparation and processing time and finally its toxicity---will the agent have any adverse (toxic) effects on either the client or CosmeCaregivers. In a great many instances the concentration of a chemical agent will determine whether it will be a disinfectant or antiseptic.

Compatibilty refers to the effects that the method or agents used for sanitizing has on the articles that are to be used for CosmeCare services. This includes corrosion or destructior, following changes in chemical composition of the article e.g. color, stability and/or changes in physical properties such as the shape, size, density, etc.

In this country there is now a greater awareness and urgency for reducing the risk of acquiring diseases from improper sanitation and hygiene e.g. many food handlers, hospital personel are now required to wear plastic gloves. Most salon owners and managers have also instituted operating procedures that require greater effort to controll the spread of microorganisms. These include use of ultraviolet (UV light) cabinets and use of chemical agents for sanitizing equipment and supplies. Two products now available for use as a surface disinfectant of metal and suitable plastic instruments and equipment used in cosmetology salons and related schools are as follows:

    *Barbicide Plus® (substitute phenates)

    Ultronics Ultracare® (N-alkyl dimethyl ethyl benzyl ammonium chloride)

It would come as no great suprise to find in the near future that new guidelines and standards for sanitation will be promulgated by most, if not all, State Regulators for use by the Salon industry and CosmeCaregivers.

COMPLETE AND RETURN THIS COUPON FOR A
FREE GIFT

✳ Bed and Pillow Protector Cover...
A Soft, Polyethylene Sheet 3 Ft. by 3 Ft.
Ideal for Several **D**ARA⁺R

Name_____

Address_____

City_____State_____Zip_____

CosmeCare And Desairology Institute
1312 Arthur Street; Dept E
Hollywood, Florida 33019

FOR FASTER SERVICE, CALL (954)929-3559; 9 am - 5 pm EST